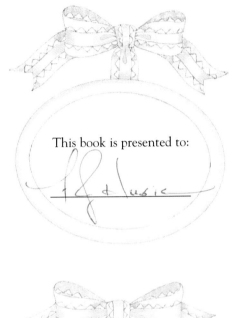

This book is presented to:

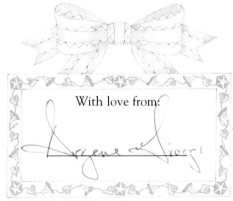

With love from:

Art Copyright Mothers' Aid Chicago Lying-in Hospital
Text copyright Regina Press
Melville, NY 11747
All rights reserved.
No part of this book may be reproduced in any form
or by any means without written permission of the Publisher.
This edition published by permission of Thomas Nelson, Inc.
ISBN: 088271-539-9
Printed in Belgium

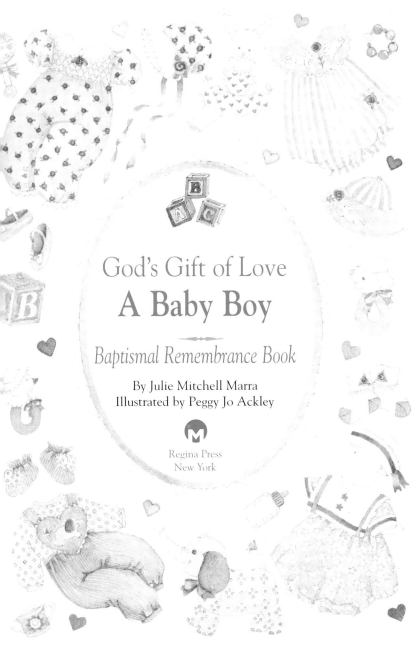

God's Gift of Love
A Baby Boy

Baptismal Remembrance Book

By Julie Mitchell Marra
Illustrated by Peggy Jo Ackley

Regina Press
New York

*D*ear Parents,
God has blessed you with a newborn son who is now the focus of your attention. Whether he is your first baby or an addition to your family, he will create a wonderful love connection. Your baby boy's birth is the beginning of a unique bonding time.

You feel so complete because this little bundle of joy brings more happiness than you could ever ask for. He is God's gift of life to you!

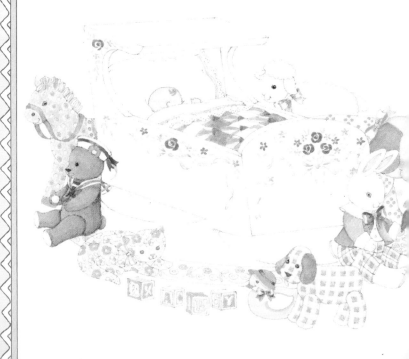

Before you know it, he will be learning and growing in grace. Remember that God will lead you and guide you in bringing up this precious little one.

As parents, you can make a unique contribution to your child's life. You create the atmosphere for your baby to learn. Your interaction with him will unfold his future. In the first few months, you may wonder if he can understand what you're telling him. He will, so tell him all that you believe and pray with him...

Our Father, who art in heaven,
hallowed be thy name;
thy kingdom come;
thy will be done, on earth as it is in heaven;
give us this day our daily bread;
and forgive us our trespasses,
as we forgive those who trespass against us;
and lead us not into temptation,
but deliver us from evil.
Amen.

Your new son may seem like a tremendous responsibility, but try to relax and savor this precious time. Cherish each moment, each smile, each frown. Someday you'll want to hold onto his hand so tight, you won't want to let go.

— *Julie Mitchell Marra*

$\mathcal{A}$ll About The Wonderful Birth of

Our Baby Boy's Name Frank F & Joseph Husic

Date of his birth September 9, 1999

Time of Birth 7:51 p.m.

Place of Birth San Francisco PCMC

Doctor Dr. David Roak

Nurses _____

Weight 8 lb.

Length 20' 3/4"

His hair color(if any) lots - Dark Brown

His eye color Dark Blue

His special characteristics Big Bright Eyes

Our family and friends who were there or sent wishes
of love Iryna Georgi, Jim & Margerie
Brewster, Millie Stake,
Abigail Baker, Karla & David
Alderma, Blanca Ramos,
Karen Caldwell, Nancy and
David
My Mom & Dad - the whole time

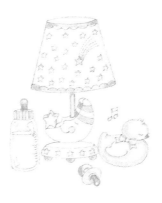

You are worthy, our Lord and God,

to receive glory and honor and power, for

you created all things and by your will

they existed and were created.

— Revelation 4:11

*O*ur Baby Boy's Baptism

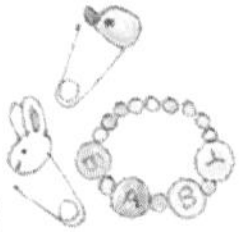

Date _Feb 4th, 2000_

Church _Sts. Peter & Paul Church - Northbo_

Priest _Father Kevin Schindler._

His godmother _Kelly Day_

His godfather _Robert Day_

How we celebrated _Service, Reception @ Carneline Room SCA_

Family and friends who attended _35 people_
attended the Service and
reception

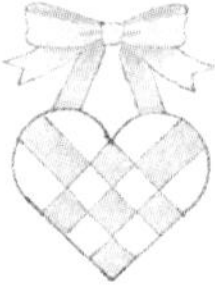

Our prayer for him _____

_____

_____

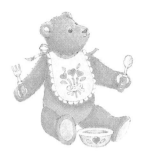

*O*ne Lord, one faith, one baptism,

one God and Father of all,

who is above all and through all

and in all.

— Ephesians 4:5-6

*T*hrough baptism, your son receives the gift of new life from God. As he is baptized, he becomes a child of God...ready to receive many blessings.

Your son is a new creation, clothed in Christ. With your help, he will learn and grow strong in faith.

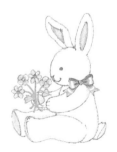

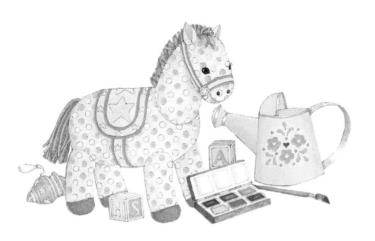

Lead him down the right path in life and, together, your family will be a beautiful example of God's love.

Your son, enlightened by Christ, is entrusted to you to keep the flame of his faith alive.

May God's love and wisdom bless your baby boy always.

Where Did You Come From?

Where did you come from, Baby dear?
Out of the everywhere into here.

Where did you get your eyes so blue?
Out of the sky as I came through.

What makes the light in them sparkle and spin?
Some of the starry spikes left in.

Where did you get that little tear?
I found it waiting when I got here.

What makes your forehead so smooth and high?
A soft hand stroked it as I went by.

What makes your cheek like a warm white rose?
I saw something better than anyone knows.

Whence that three-corner'd smile of bliss?
Three angels gave me at once a kiss.

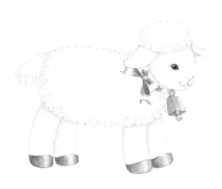

Where did you get this pearly ear?
God spoke, and it came out to hear.

Where did you get those arms and hands?
Love made itself into hooks and bands.

Feet, whence did you come, you darling things?
From the same box as cherubs wings.

How did they all come just to be you?
God thought of me, and so I grew.

But how did you come to us, you dear?
God thought of you, and so I am here.

— *George MacDonald*

A Cradle Song

Sweet dreams form a shade,
O'er my lovely infant's head.
Sweet dreams of pleasant streams,
By happy silent moony beams.

Sweet sleep with soft down,
Weave thy brows an infant crown.
Sweet sleep Angel mild,
Hover o'er my happy child.

Sweet smiles in the night,
Hover over my delight.
Sweet smiles, Mother's smiles,
All the livelong might beguiles.

Sweet moans, dovelike sighs,
Chase not slumber from thy eyes.
Sweet moans, sweeter smiles,
All the dovelike moans beguiles.

Sleep, sleep happy child.
All creation slept and smil'd.
Sleep, sleep, happy sleep,
While o'er you your mother weep.

Sweet babe in your face,
Holy image I can trace.
Sweet babe once like thee,
Your maker lay and wept for me,

Wept for me, for you, for all,
When he was an infant small.
Thou his image ever see,
Heavenly smiles on you;

Smiles on you, on me, on all,
Who become an infant small,
Infant smiles are his own smiles,
Heaven & earth to peace beguiles.

— *William Blake*

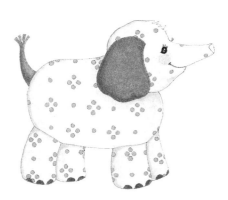

O, King of the Tree of Life,

The blossoms on your branches are your people,
The singing birds are your angels,
The whispering breeze is your Spirit.

O, King of the Tree of Life,
May the blossoms bring forth the sweetest fruit,
May the birds sing out the highest praise
May your Spirit cover all with his gentle breath.

— *Celtic Prayer*

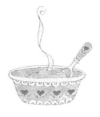

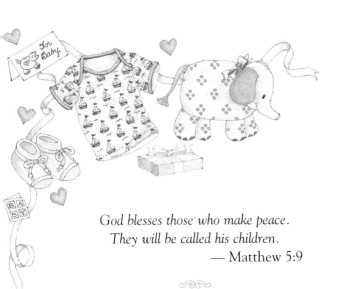

God blesses those who make peace.
They will be called his children.
— Matthew 5:9

✧

I lift up this newborn child to you.
You brought it to birth, you gave it life.
This child is a fresh bud on an ancient tree,
A new member of an old family.
May this fresh bud blossom.
May this child grow up strong and righteous.
— *Margery Kempe*

✧

Good people live right and God blesses
the children who follow their example.
— Proverbs 20:7

Mother's Heart

When first you camest, gentle, shy, and fond,
My eldest born, first hope, and dearest treasure,
My heart received you with a joy beyond
All that it yet had felt of earthly pleasure.
— *Caroline E. Norton*

Where we love is home,
Home where our feet may leave,
But not our hearts.
— *Oliver Wendell Holmes*

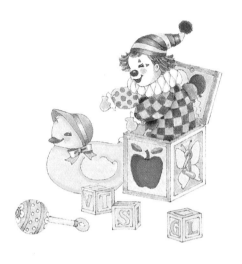

Let the little children come to me,
Do not stop them;
for it is to such as these
that the kingdom of God belongs.
— Mark 10:14

$\mathcal{B}$arefoot Boy

Blessings on you, little man,
Barefoot boy, with cheek of tan!
With your turned-up pantaloons,
And your merry whistled tunes;
With your red lips, redder still,
Kissed by strawberries on the hill;
With the sunshine on your face,
Through your torn brim's jaunty grace:
from my heart I give you joy;
I was once a barefoot boy!
Cheerily, then, my little man,
Live and laugh, as boyhood can...
Ah! That you could know your joy,
Ere it passes, Barefoot Boy!

— *John Greenleaf Whittier*

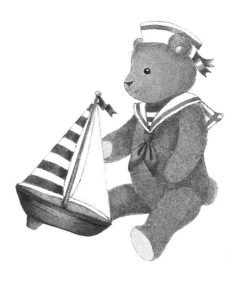

The mystery that has been hidden
throughout the ages and generations
but has now been revealed
to his saints...which is Christ in you,
the hope of glory.

— Colossians 1:26-27

*T*he Soul of Your Child

The soul of your child is the loveliest flower
That grows in the garden of God.
Its climb is from weakness to knowledge and power
To the sky from the clay to the clod.
To beauty and sweetness it grows under care.
Neglected, 'tis ragged and wild.
'Tis a plant that is tender, but wondrously rare.
The sweet wistful soul of a child.
Be tender, O Gardner, and give it its share
Of moisture, of warmth and of light,
And let it not lack for the painstaking care
To protect it from frost and from blight.
A glad day will come when its bloom shall unfold,
It will seem that an angel has smiled
Reflecting a beauty and sweetness untold
In the sensitive soul of your child.

— *Author Unknown*

Perfect Home

The man is the brace and ceiling
of his house
He is the straight walls rising
from the earth.
The woman is the golden glow
of lamps,
The firelight on a hearth.
A man to the home is
a sheltering roof,
A wind break, refuge from
storm and rain.
A woman is the warm, bright
scarlet flower
Beyond the window pane.
Their children are the sun and
rays that sweep
Through open doors, a blessed
thing so good.
Trinity on earth that makes a
"home"
Where once a mere
house stood.

— *Emery Petho*

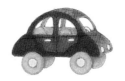

$\mathcal{M}$other's Hope

Is there, when the winds are singing
In the happy summer time,
When the raptured air is ringing
With the Earth's music heavenward spring,
Forest chirp and village chime.

Is there, of the sounds that float
Unsighingly, a single note
Half so sweet, and clear, and wild,
As the laughter of a child?
— *Laman Blanchard*

Rock Me to Sleep, Mother

Clasped to your heart in a loving embrace,
With your light lashes just sweeping my face,
Never hereafter to wake or to weep;
Rock me to sleep, Mother, rock me to sleep.

— *Elizabeth Chase Akers*

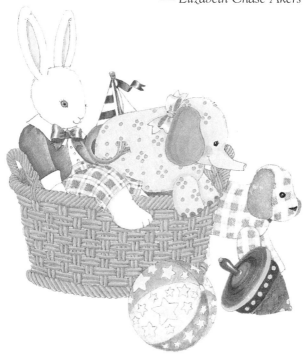

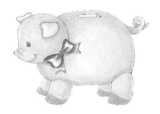

If your child lives with tolerance,
he learns to be patient.
If your child lives with praise,
he learns to be appreciative.
If your child lives with acceptance
he learns to love.
If your child lives with approval
he learns to like himself.
If your child lives with recognition
he learns it is good to have a goal.
If your child lives with fairness
he learns what justice is.
If your child lives with honesty
he learns what truth is.
If your child lives with security
he learns to have faith in himself
and those about him.
If your child lives with friendliness
he learns the world is a nice place in
which to live...
— *Author Unknown*

Honor your father and your mother,
so that your days may be long
in the land that the Lord your God
is giving you.

— Exodus 20:12

Hear my child your father's instruction
and do not reject your mother's teaching;
for they are as a fair garland for your head
and pendants for your neck.

— Proverbs 1:8-9

Loving a Little Boy

Loving a little boy is a quicksilver thing.

He will escape the circling of an arm,
resent the smoothing of his hair's dark wing,
Scorn a suggestion he might come to harm.

But there is a time of day, or perhaps of night,
When weary of play, reluctant yet to go
Stairward, the lanterns in his eyes less bright,
he may pause with a nonchalant step and slow
beside his mother's chair, or rest awhile
Against her knee, without the airs he wore,
But bay-soft and with the secret smile
Of one who deals with fairies and their lore.

This is the moment burning like an ember,
That she will never forget, or he remember.

— *Eleanor A. Chaffee*

*C*radle Song

Who can tell me what a baby thinks?
Who can follow the gossamer links
By which the mankind manikin feels his way
Out from the shore of the great unknown,
Blind, and wailing, and alone,
Into the light of day?

— *Josiah Gilbert Holland*

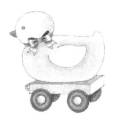

*In the fear of the Lord
one has strong confidence
and one's children will have a refuge.*

— Proverbs 14:26-27

*D*ear God,

Help me to show my son Your heart of compassion. Show him contentment with the things that You give. Instill in me the insight to teach my child the important lessons in life.

Give me the courage to set an example of what is right and wrong; and help my son to walk in the right path following You.

I pray my son will know Your Word to be true. May he find peace and the answers in life in Your Word. Then may he spread Your loving message.

Show me how to lead him in Your special plan for his life.

Amen

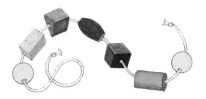

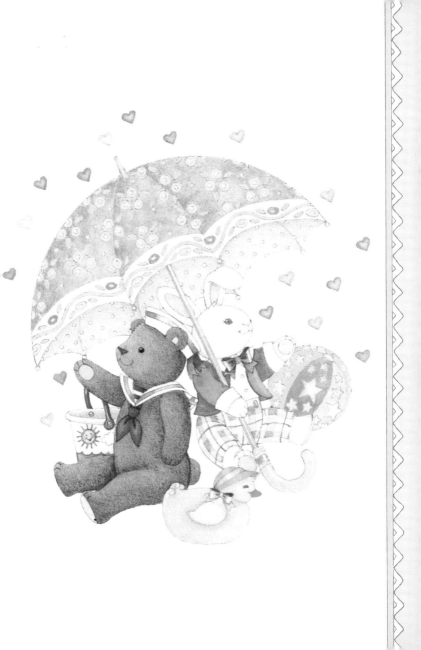

Designed by Millicent Iacono

Typeset in Goudy, Caslon Titling
and Caslon Swash

PRINTED IN BELGIUM BY

INTERNATIONAL BOOK PRODUCTION